…In Faith

Praying, Trusting, Believing, Conceiving,
Faith Rewarded®

Dr. Latara O. Lampkin

Faith Rewarded® series

For we are saved by hope: but hope that is seen is not hope: for what a man seeth, why doth he yet hope for?
Romans 8:24

In Faith

© 2019
All rights reserved. Except for the brief quotations used in reviews, articles, or other media, no part of this book may be reproduced or transmitted in any form or by any means, electronic or mechanical, including photocopying, recording, or by information storage or retrieval system, without the express, written consent of the authors.

Scriptures taken from the New King James Version®. Copyright © 1982 by Thomas Nelson. Used by permission. All rights reserved.

Scripture marked NAS is taken from the NEW AMERICAN STANDARD (NAS): Scripture taken from the NEW AMERICAN STANDARD BIBLE®, copyright© 1960, 1962, 1963, 1968, 1971, 1972, 1973, 1975, 1977, 1995 by The Lockman Foundation. Used by permission.

Cover Design/Layout: Nathan Archer
Editor: Katie Lowery

ISBN: 978-1-7339625-0-6

This book is a tribute to our son, Marcus M. Lampkin Jr., who, through the grace of God, was conceived July 2005. He entered the world on March 16, 2006. Marcus Jr.'s conception is evidence of God's willingness to honor our prayers and our faith in him.

We thank God for the blessing and honored responsibility that he has bestowed upon us in parenting our son. Marcus is truly a manifestation of his works and ability to do all things, should we just believe.

Table of Contents

Introduction 6

Chapter One – Stepping into the Faith Zone ... 10

Chapter Two – Honor of Faith 17

Chapter Three – Walking in Faith 23

Chapter Four – Test of Faith 27

Chapter Five – Measure of Faith 31

Chapter Six – A Journey of Faith 37

Chapter Seven – Stepping out on Faith 45

Chapter Eight – Sustaining Faith 49

Afterword 51

Introduction

For this child I prayed; and the Lord hath given me my petition which I asked of him.
(1 Samuel 1:27)

I have often heard ministers say, "Prayer is one of the greatest privileges we have as God's children." I have come to know that this is, indeed, true. It is through our prayers that we really connect with God – it is our direct connection to him. I believe this is why we teach children how to pray at an early age, even before they can fully understand the words or meaning behind the prayer. Teaching our children to pray gives us peace of mind that they have a source for comfort and guidance, even when they cannot connect with us. As a young child, I was taught the Our Father prayer. Admittedly, it was not until I was much older that I really understood the words, and most importantly, the power of those words and how they would connect me with the Father.

> *Our Father, which art in heaven, Hallowed be thy name, thy kingdom come, thy will be done, on earth as it is in heaven. Give us this day our daily bread...* (Matthew 6:9)

Many of us have recited this prayer countless times. It has become a ritual for some of us. Some would argue that ritualistic prayers can serve a purpose, but I am not convinced. We are reminded in Matthew 6:7 that *"when we pray, we are not to use vain repetitions."* In fact, the entire sixth chapter of Matthew provides direction on issues surrounding prayer. While I wouldn't presume to add anything to the word of God on the matter, I will say that deeply embedded in the scripture is the importance of using prayer to connect to our Father, not just to meet our needs but to strengthen our relationship and connection to him.

Prayer is more than a set of ritualistic words that we mumble before we eat, sleep, or begin our day. They are also more than what I call "crisis prayers." Most of us have needed to plead in prayer at one point or another: "Oh my God, I need you now because…" You are quite fortunate if you have never had to finish that sentence. I have pleaded with God many times over. As recording artist Erica Campbell eloquently puts it, sometimes we simply must call out for "Help!"

I am in constant communication with God, and this prayerful relationship has been essential to helping me navigate life. I petition the Lord in prayer about all things, big and small. I have prayed, "Lord, please direct my path as I make this life-changing decision." I have also prayed, "Lord, help me find a parking space. I am so late for this meeting!"

I have taken this approach because based on my relationship with the Lord, I know that he *"is able to do exceedingly above all that I can ask or think…"* (Ephesians 3:20). I am confident that he will answer my prayers, as he has done time and time again. I turn to consultation with God before all major decisions and in times of crisis or change.

In 2005, I went into consultation with God and was granted one of the most amazing miracles in my life: the conception of our son. This book is our attempt to follow God's direction and minister to those who are struggling with having faith that God will grant their prayers to become parents. Ordinarily, we are very private people, so sharing our story was a difficult choice, but we have felt directed by God to share our testimony. We are sharing our journey because we know that it's easy to feel alone in times of struggle, when the truth is that many others are traveling the same road. There is no need to take this journey in complete isolation. You are not alone. Even when you are physically alone and you feel that you have no one to confide in, you can turn to God. God is always there.

We petition you to seek God diligently and faithfully. Know that others have come before you and have, indeed, had their prayers answered. We wholeheartedly believe that as you "*delight thyself in the Lord; he shall give you the desires of your heart*" (Psalms 37:4). We would like to restore the faith and hope lost during your journey, and we pray that through our testimony you will be encouraged to believe and trust that God will honor your diligence and faith. Jesus said, "*All things are possible for one who believes*" (Mark 9:23).

I believe that we must always position ourselves to receive a word. We pray that you will position yourself to receive our testimony. It is a testament to our relationship with our Father, your Father, and to his faithfulness in answering our prayers. Finally, we pray that your prayers will also be answered.

Chapter One

Stepping into the Faith Zone
A Mother's Prayer

Children are a heritage from the Lord, the fruit of the womb, a reward. (Psalm 127:3)

One of the most rewarding blessings is the gift of a child. In fact, the creation of life and the birth of children are among God's greatest gifts.

It is through parenting that we have the privilege and opportunity to create and shape the life of another human being. As parents, we are given a gift that hopefully keeps giving. We are entrusted with the life of another individual who will make a mark on the world, whatever that mark might be. For some of us, parenting can be the gift of a second chance, but for all of us, parenthood offers the gift of unconditional love.

If we are not careful we can miss out on the gift if it does not arrive in the packaging we expect or prefer. When it came to having children, that perfect packaging for me was timing. My desire to have children was balanced with my career goals. I was focused, driven, and proud of my success and hard work. So, the timing had to be just right or I believed that the gift would not be perfect.

I proudly ignored the annoying questions and comments that many newlyweds hear. "When are you going to have a baby?" "Now that you are married, you can start your family!" "What are you waiting for?" It became so predictable that I had to mentally prepare for the onslaught of questions at family gatherings. In speaking with a colleague who struggled with infertility prior to having her son, I learned that the "dreaded questions" are actually quite common.

Understandingly, the possibility of a new baby in the family warrants asking or encouraging, particularly from prospective grandparents. A new baby is always the center of attention at any family gathering and is a favorite topic of conversation in general. Most of us smile at the sight of new baby, typically viewing them as special gifts.

As newlyweds, however, we were more excited about being married and spending countless hours just being with each other. We took to heart the adage that "after a baby, your life is never the same." So, for years, we ignored the questions and remarks, cherished our time together, and planned for the "perfect time." Little did we know that it would not be in our timing, but in God's timing that our gift would be manifested.

After four years of marriage, Marcus and I, both avid planners, began to plan for our first child. We reviewed our financial plans, insurance plans, medical plans – every detail we could imagine was reviewed and adjusted accordingly. The planning was endless. We wanted to make sure that we had covered all the bases, knowing that this would be one of the most important decisions of our lives. We would later be reminded that we could make our own plans, but the counsel of the Lord would stand (Proverbs 19:21, NAS).

I threw out my contraceptives and proceeded to the doctor for a full physical. In the office of a trusted gynecologist, we received the heartbreaking news. We were informed that it was very unlikely that I would be able to conceive without medical intervention. The reason: fibroid tumors. I had been aware of them for years, but they had never been an issue before.

Marcus and I looked into each other's eyes, saddened but eager to hear our options. A friend once explained it as human nature. "We want most what we are told we cannot have." I guess in our case, it was true, because in that moment we wanted a baby more than ever. Every maternal and paternal instinct that we had was immediately activated.

We left the office with a stack of literature on fibroids and an appointment with a fertility specialist. My doctor's words still echoed in my head. "It is very unlikely that you will be able to conceive without medical intervention. Without the surgical removal of the fibroid tumors blocking the passage of the fallopian tubes, you will not be able to conceive." As a graduate student in a doctoral program, major surgery just was not feasible. It was not in our carefully constructed plan, so it was not an option. Although I had been hearing what my doctor was saying, I was not actively listening.

As we drove home, we decided that we would research the medical procedures available to address the fibroids, and would at least have an initial consultation with the fertility specialist. Over a six-month period, I underwent several tests and began to have increased physical discomfort. After reviewing our options, we decided to proceed with the myomectomy, one of the most complex surgical procedures for removing the fibroids. During this stressful time, I began to pray. I am not talking about a morning or nightly ritual prayer, but a purposeful prayer – a direct request! In fact, I began to pray to God the first day we met with my doctor. Within only a few days, I heard a sermon from one of my now-favorite pastors, Joel Osteen. He posed the question: "Whose report will you believe? Will you believe God or will you believe the negative reports? …Step over into the Faith Zone!"

I also searched the scriptures of the New King James Bible. I started carrying a small notepad in my purse, where I would jot down passages that spoke to me. I was led to the following scriptures and wrote:

> Father, I declare that I will conceive and give birth to a healthy child!

> *And the angel came in unto her and said, Hail, thou that art highly favored, the Lord is with thee: blessed art thou among women.*
> *And the angel said unto her, Fear not (Latara); for thou has found favor in God.*

And behold, thou shalt conceive in thy womb, and bring forth a son... and shalt call his name (Myles). (Luke 1:28; 20-31)

To address the fibroids, I searched the Bible for healing scriptures. I wrote:

Have mercy upon me, O Lord; for I am weak: O Lord, heal me; for my bones are weak. (Psalms 6:2)

But he was wounded for our transgression, he was bruised for our inequities: the chastisement of our peace was upon him; and with his stripes we are healed. (Isaiah 53:5)

And the prayer of faith shall save the sick, and the Lord shall raise him up; and if he have committed sins, they shall be forgiven him.
Confess your faults one to another, and pray one for another that you may be healed. The effectual fervent prayer of the righteous man availath much. (James 5:15-16)

And Jesus saith unto him, I will come and heal him. (Matthew 8:7)

Finally, I found a passage that would come to mean more to me than words can express. It wasn't until later that I thought, "Perhaps I was too specific." I included:

And she (Latara) shall bring forth a son… (Matthew 1:21)

I prayed every day and read the scriptures sometimes two or three times a day. Whenever I needed encouragement, I read the scriptures in my notebook. I prayed and I read. I read and I prayed. Most of all, I believed with all my heart that God would grant my request.

Chapter Two

Honor of Faith

And blessed is she that believed: for there shall be a performance of those things which were told to her. (Luke 1:45)

For he that is mighty hath done to me great things; and holy is his name. (Luke 1:49)

The journey to the conception of our son began with a belief that God would surely hear and grant our petition. In fact, I believed he would answer our prayer despite the long odds. In addition to my medical condition, my husband and I were living in two different states thanks to a recent job opportunity. We were miles apart (1,173 miles, to be exact), yet I was asking God to help us conceive a child when we would only see each other for fewer than six days a month for the next six months. While this might seem like another barrier, I wholeheartedly believe that God created a situation that would serve two purposes. First and foremost, our separation would enable us to develop even closer relationships with God. Second, we would have an even more powerful testimony.

During these six months, I had many moments of silence, particularly in the evenings. My solitude gave me the chance to sit still and experience a new level of mindfulness. I was also praying often and with intention. Not only was I diligent in prayer and reflection, but frankly, some evenings there was just no one else to talk to. So, I talked to God. He had purposefully placed me in a position to reflect and hear his voice.

My family, friends, and colleagues can attest to the fact that I am rarely at a loss for words. I can hold a complete conversation all by myself. As an only child for nineteen years, I was often required to entertain myself. This likely also explains my contentment with being with myself and embracing silence. I truly welcomed the quiet time and the opportunity to develop a better relationship with God. I talked and I talked and I talked. For one of the first times in my life, I actually waited for an answer or some type of confirmation. During each of our conversations, I reminded him of my desire to be a mother, and of how busy I was with school. I simply could not manage to be out for six weeks to recover from surgery, even if it meant an increased chance to conceive.

I was resolute and unwavering for months.

Day after day, month after month, I had the same conversation with God. Eventually, I began to question my insistence to conceive without medical intervention. Was I like the stranded man in the parable who drowned because he turned away all the help that came his way? Caught on his roof amid rising floodwaters, the man declined help from several boats and a helicopter, insistent that God would save him. When the waters swept him away and he drowned, he went to heaven and asked God why he had not come to his aid. God replied, "I sent you a rowboat. You did not get in." Was I like this man, refusing the solution that God was granting me? This story influenced my decision to at least consider surgery as an option. I later concluded that perhaps God was directing me to have the medical procedure. Maybe the surgery was the provision that he was making so that he could honor my request.

Ultimately, my husband and I decided to have the fibroids surgically removed. With the upcoming surgery, we would be closer to becoming parents, but we decided to keep the entire process to ourselves. I wanted to respond to the dreaded question with an update on our progress, but instead, I kept quiet and felt an inward confidence in knowing that I had finally heard God and was open to the provision he had provided us to conceive and become a family.

The week leading up to the surgery was filled with lots of preparation and planning. We made sure that our medical leave was arranged, and we completed all the paperwork for the pre-op visit on Tuesday. Yet, on Sunday night, just a few days before the pre-op appointment, I decided to throw a pregnancy test in the cart while shopping. I could not even guess how many pregnancy tests I took over that six-month period, even when there was no indication that there was a chance of conception. Nonetheless, on that Sunday evening, I placed the test in the cart as I had done so many times before. My husband sighed and said, "Here we go again. The doctor said that you must have the surgery before we'll have a chance." I replied, "Let's just see."

Later that evening, after getting settled in for the night, I snuck into the bathroom to take the pregnancy test. I did my routine of praying and reading the scriptures in my notepad before opening the test. Despite being convinced that maybe the surgery was God's provision for conception, I still knew that through him, anything was possible. Just five days before surgery, I was still trusting God to hear my initial request.

Even in the eleventh hour, even when there does not appear to be a chance, God can and will answer your prayer. In fact, his blessing is magnified when it seems that all hope is lost. I had a pre-op appointment in two days and was planning to have a myomectomy at the end of that week, and yet, I still had faith. I think back now and laugh at the fact that I would have had faith right until the moment I was put under anesthesia.

I took the test. Two red lines. Pregnant. I sat down and stared at the positive test for at least five minutes before yelling to my husband. He came and was in total disbelief. He assumed that I was joking and insisted that I take another test. Once again, there were two lines, and this time, I had a witness. We were so excited! We hugged, kissed, and vowed not to tell anyone before we had official results from the doctor. Of course I was going to adhere to this, right?

My husband went back to doing his thing around the house, and I immediately called my dear friend and shared the exciting news, breaking the vow of secrecy I'd made only moments before. In the same breath, I explained that I was not supposed to be telling anyone yet. My friend and I could not contain ourselves. We cheered, we prayed, we cried, we praised God, all in a whisper. Next, I called my mom. I tried to keep the news to myself, but I just couldn't.

Genesis 16:11 states, *"And the angel of the Lord said unto her, Behold, thou art with child and shalt bear a son, and shalt call his name Ishmael; because the LORD hath heard thy affliction."* I was convinced that God had heard my prayers, and despite my affliction, had granted my request. Not only had he answered my prayers, but his timing was perfect. In 2 Samuel 22:31, we are reminded that, *"As for God, his way is perfect; the word of the LORD is tried: he is a buckler to all them that trust in him."* Two months earlier, my mom had lost her best friend of more than 30 years. I had the opportunity to share some news with her that had come only because of my trust in God. Instead of preparing for surgery, we were preparing for a baby. This was, indeed, a happy time. Little did we know that we would need to continue to trust him.

Chapter Three

Walking in Faith
The Road Less Traveled?

Again, I say unto you, That if two of you shall agree on earth as touching any thing that they shall ask, it shall be done for them of my Father which is in heaven. (Matthew 18:19)

We were certainly excited about Marcus' conception, but the road to get there had been lonely. Infertility is not isolated to only an unlucky few. The American Society of Reproductive Medicine reports that more than six million people, approximately ten percent of individuals of reproductive age, suffer from infertility. Not only is infertility widespread, but there are over one hundred reported conditions that may contribute to or cause infertility in both men and women. In my case, the root cause was leiomyomas or myomas, commonly known as fibroid tumors, another common condition for women.

If infertility is such a common issue, why do we feel alone on this journey? It's so easy to let yourself believe that you are the only one struggling with fertility issues, but the truth is that one in eight couples have trouble getting or staying pregnant. The odds are good that you know at least one person who has walked the same path. So why is infertility so lonely?

I certainly don't know the answer to this question for all women who have dealt with infertility. There is not one single answer. There are multiple factors that influence our thinking about and experiences with dealing with issues of infertility. For me, the notion of preparing to have a baby was a private issue. Some women feel ashamed that they cannot conceive, and others feel that sex in general is a private topic. This was not the case for me. I do not share personal matters, and it was simply nobody's business. Even though I didn't want to share our struggles publicly, carrying the weight alone can take an emotional and sometimes physical toll. I had no one with whom to share the pain or fear of imperfection, the fear of the unknown, and even the fear of not being able to deal with the stress.

Eventually, keeping our struggle to myself was no longer an option. I realized that there were others who really needed someone to talk to, someone to empathize with them, someone who was walking the same path. After two miscarriages, one of my dear friends shared, "What do people say? What *can* they say? They mean well, but if it hasn't happened to them, they can never understand." Another friend said, "It is when you cannot have something that you want it the most." Finally, a colleague explained, "Motherhood is one of the many things that define a woman. Not at least having the option can somehow make you feel like less of a woman." Despite the loving support of their husbands, who tried to understand and who clearly experienced some of the same fears, each of these women felt compelled to deal with the issue alone.

When we face an issue that we believe no one else can possibly understand, we try to put on a brave face and shoulder the weight privately. It is during these times that we must push ourselves to do the absolute opposite. In fact, we should feel comforted to know that "*if two shall agree on earth as touching anything that they shall ask, it shall be done for them of my Father which is in heaven. For where two or three are gathered in my name, there am I in the midst of them*" (Matthew 18:19-20). God encourages us to find others who can support us in our time of need. We are not traveling the road alone. When the night seems darkest, we should seek out and rely on our prayer warriors to help us to pray our way through! We are told that we should *"pray one for another [...] and the effectual prayer of the righteous availeth much"* (James 5:16). I am so grateful for the many prayer warriors who became our "faith warriors." They embraced and surrounded us during our time of need. Some of these same generous people helped pray Marcus into existence, others prayed for his continued existence.

Chapter Four

Test of Faith

...yet will I trust in him. (Job 13:15)

The road to delivery was long and stressful. Due to the common complications associated with fibroids, I was placed on bedrest within the first two months of the pregnancy. Later, on the day of our baby shower in south Florida, the baby repositioned and I went into premature labor, two months early.

I encountered many difficulties with conceiving and carrying our child, but I found comfort in the story of Elisabeth and Mary. Luke 1:44 reminds us that *"with God nothing shall be impossible."* Given the issues associated with conception, Elisabeth must have had some concerns about the health of her unborn baby. In this case, I am reminded of an interaction between Mary and Elisabeth. Mary *"entered into the house of Zacharias, and saluted Elisabeth. When Elisabeth heard the salutation of Mary, the babe leaped in her womb; and Elisabeth was filled with the Holy Ghost."* Her baby's movement must have been confirmation to Elisabeth that all was well. I thought of this story as my baby repositioned himself and took it as confirmation that there was, indeed, life inside what had been considered a barren womb.

After the south Florida scare and several trips to the ER for false alarms, my *"full time came that I should deliver; and I brought forth (my) son"* (Luke 1:57). Marcus M. Lampkin Jr. graced us with his presence on March 16, 2006. Yes, 3:16. I had declared that we would call our son Myles, and as we got closer to the due date, we began to talk to baby Myles and call him by name. When she met our son for the first time, my mom asked, "What will you name him?" Without missing a beat, my husband, Marcus, responded, "Marcus Lampkin Jr." Hence, baby Myles became MJ.

Marcus Lampkin Jr. brought a new joy to our lives that only a baby can. The wonder of parenting was extraordinary. We loved every bit and cherished every day with our new blessing. During the week of Thanksgiving 2006, however, that joy dimmed.

Marcus Jr. began to exhibit cold-like symptoms. As first-time parents, we immediately took him to see the doctor, who requested blood work. We were unable to reach our pediatrician's office for the results before traveling for the holiday, but I later received a message that I should call back on Monday because "something was wrong with Marcus' blood work." I received this information on a Tuesday, which meant an agonizing five-day wait before we would know what was wrong. Waiting was simply not an option, not when something was wrong with my child. I called the office repeatedly, and finally, I reached a nurse who insisted that I would need to speak directly to the doctor. I sat in my car, in the parking lot of a department store, to brace myself for the news that would change my life as I had known it as a mother.

I finally got my son's doctor on the phone, and she said, "Yes, the baby's blood work was abnormal. It's probably related to his sickle cell. His counts were so low that he will likely need a blood transfusion." My heart fell into my stomach. I gasped and immediately asked, "*What* sickle cell?"

After an awkward pause, Marcus' pediatrician explained that a diagnosis was made at his birth, but we were never informed. She then gave me instructions for his care for the next few days. I heard what she was saying, but I was not really listening. I sat in that parking lot for an hour, in shock and sadness, before I called my husband to explain the situation.

I attempted to explain something that I still didn't understand myself. I made the calls to arrange the medication and care that my son needed, which took more than five hours. As I took care of business, I also tried to process and digest the startling news. My son was diagnosed with a chronic illness. Despite a few tearful outbursts, I did not have time to cope with the complexity of what this really meant, and I had no idea what lay ahead. I simply asked in agony, "Lord, why me?"

Chapter Five

Measure of Faith
The Purpose of His Coming and God's Calling

And we know that all things work together for good to them that love God, to them who are called according to his purpose. (Romans 8:28)

Why me? Most of us can recall a point in our lives that we have asked this question. Those of you who have been steadfast in your faith and have trusted in God without ever wavering, you have been blessed! It is so easy, when consumed by our circumstances, to waver in our faith. When you find yourself asking, "Lord, why me," know that there is an answer to this question: for God's purpose.

God's purpose was revealed to me on two separate occasions. I first understood God's purpose during a discussion with my husband, and again when hearing a story from another mother of a chronically ill child.

When talking with my husband, ever the realist, I asked that same old question again. Overcome with the frustration of it all, I demanded, "Why us? Why me?" My husband responded, "Why not you?" While his words were not comforting, they were profound.

A few weeks later, I received a similar response to my question. A story on the radio caught my attention while I drove home. I missed the beginning of the story, but I know it was in God's perfect timing.

The narrator told the story of a woman with an ill child. The mother felt helpless as she watched her child suffer for years. One day she broke down and cried, "Lord, why me? Why would you place me in such a helpless state? You can't imagine how it feels to see your child suffering." As she wallowed in her pain, the mother had a revelation. *"For God so loved the world that he gave his only begotten son"* (John 3:16). Giving the ultimate sacrifice, God and Mary had indeed witnessed their son suffer. The mother began to cry as she was reminded how God had watched his only son hang on the cross to give us the gift of life.

Tears began to stream down my face like the mother in the story. I, too, had forgotten. I immediately asked God for forgiveness. "Father, forgive me! You know firsthand what I am going through. Like me, you have witnessed the suffering of your only son."

I made a conscious effort to stop complaining and instead to ask for help to sustain me through the situation. I prayed, *"Thou has been my help. Leave me not; neither forsake me"* (Psalms 27:9).

This became a recurring prayer. I turned to it for comfort during the many hours and days of my son's pain crises and other complications associated with his illness.

I cried for another hour, thanking God for this purposeful experience. Hearing this story only weeks after my son's diagnosis, I knew that this was an ordained appointment. With this understanding, I remembered the words of a dear friend: "Everything is purposeful." It is during the "difficult, purposeful experiences" that our faith can truly be measured.

I have come to believe that everything is indeed purposeful. I often say that God gives "special gifts" to good stewards. I liken my son and his illness to a gift. For those caring for chronically ill children, the stress and burden may occasionally make you question this claim.

The stress can strain your health, your resources, and sometimes even your relationships. Yet, everything is purposeful.

Knowing that there is purpose to be found in every situation, remember to *"Give thanks unto the Lord; for he is good; his mercy endureth forever"* (Psalms 106:1). If not for anything else, we can thank God for our children. They are blessings!

I cannot say that I have never questioned the magnitude of the blessing, or if, in fact, my son's birth was a blessing at all. After one of the early hospital visits in which Marcus was treated for a sickle cell crisis, I drove home exhausted. We were going on our fifth day in the hospital and we were all tired. I called a friend to give her an update on Marcus Jr.'s status and hopefully find some support.

I began the conversation with the normal reassurances that Marcus Jr. was getting progressively better and that Marcus and I were doing fine. Despite the gravity of his condition, our family and friends typically noticed our attempts to limit their concerns and rarely pried. My friend picked up on my attempt to downplay the magnitude of my worry and fear, but chose to lovingly confront me. She said, "The enemy would have you believe that your blessing is indeed a burden."

I was so taken aback that I had to pull to the side of the road. This had become a routine, pulling over to digest information related to my son's medical condition. I had to process what she was saying. My son, a burden? Yes, the four hospital stays in the past three months had weighed on us tremendously. Yes, sitting in intensive care in a daze for days as doctors discussed "routine" procedures from which major complications could arise was taxing. However, it was something that we had simply accepted as a way of life, at least for our lives. It was our normal. But a burden? Of course not.

Yet, in the back of my mind, I admitted that the fear of the unknown, the unexpected crises, and the financial load of a thousand dollars in co-pays within two months were, indeed, burdens. The weight of these burdens can destroy families. Yet, my son, himself, was not a burden. He was, and is, a gift!

Again, I say God knew! He gave us this "special gift" because he knew that we would be good stewards. He knew that we would not only be an advocate for our child but for other children as well. We would be advocates for the cause. So, he called us to serve.

There are many motivations to serve. Some are innately altruistic, while other people hear God's calling. Some need a little push, waiting for God's explicit direction to serve. Just think of all the people whose personal circumstances purposed them to channel their resources, influence, time, and energy to bring awareness or to advocate for a cause that they would not have otherwise. These people likely would never have championed these causes if the situation had not affected them personally, if it had not hit home. It took a "crisis." In our case, it was a sickle cell crisis.

For families like ours, who have been blessed with these special children, we pray that you never feel as though your gift is a burden. Instead, we pray that you accept that God calls us in different ways and that this is just part of your calling.

I also encourage you to not only continue to talk and petition God along this journey for your heart's desire, but to also take time to listen. It is through hearing God's voice that we will be positioned and equipped to carry out the purpose for which we have been called.

Chapter Six

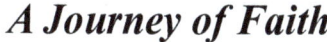

A Journey of Faith

Not by might, nor by power, but by my spirit, saith the LORD of hosts. (Zechariah 4:6)

During the early years of Marcus Jr.'s medical issues, we continued to receive confirmation that this was a predestined journey. During one of our early visits to the pediatric hospital, we received another reminder.

As I sat in the waiting room of the hospital's pediatric hematology and oncology clinic, I was surrounded by children and parents in situations very similar to our own. Some parents sat quietly with blank stares and concerned faces, and others attempted to offer comfort with a kind smile. They all had the "I know what you are going through" look. Their children, with hairless heads and wide smiles, were simply on a doctor's visit, going through familiar procedures. Their normal was also our normal.

It was during one of these visits that I had the honor and pleasure of meeting a boy I will refer to as Marshall. Marshall's bald head and the port in his arm clearly identified him as a cancer patient. If not for his outward appearance, no one would have known that he was ill. With a smile, Marshall greeted one of the doctors and casually explained that he was, "just here to get my chemo." Marshall's frankness and the normality of this experience was heartbreaking. Yet, witnessing this interaction between a child and his doctor was also very encouraging. Despite his difficult situation, Marshall was doing his best to wear a smile and operate business as usual. He was a normal three-year-old boy, just living.

I share the story about Marshall for two reasons. First, Marshall's positive attitude was an inspiration. Second, as I wandered the halls of the pediatric intensive care unit where my own son would receive treatment, Marshall reminded me that I was not alone.

I wish I could say that the feelings of isolation and weariness of caring for a child with a chronic illness never resurfaced, but that would not be true. I sometimes feel lonely. I feel overwhelmed. I feel helpless. I am angry. I feel like no one understands. I am often anxious. Over the years, I have posed that old question more than once: Why me? Why my child? The only difference is that now it's a rhetorical question.

It has been a long journey. For the first seven years of Marcus' life, we were in the hospital at least four or five times per year, sometimes for weeks at a time. We did have a reprieve; for a three-year period, he was only hospitalized once or twice a year. In 2017 and 2018, he was admitted twice, but visited the emergency room several times and averaged two to three crises per year. Each crisis lasts for three to ten days and takes a toll on Marcus Jr.'s body and our family's emotional well-being. After being in pain for several days, Marcus Jr. starts asking us why it hurts so badly or why he has sickle cell anemia. These are often rhetorical questions, but I wish I had an answer for him. Our response has remained relatively consistent, as have our feelings of helplessness.

Over the years, our family, friends, and co-workers have been genuinely concerned and offered to help. It is always comforting, but there is usually nothing they can do. We have not known how to accept help, or even wanted to accept it. We don't want to overburden family and friends, especially emotionally. This is our normal. Instead, we have cast our burdens onto the Lord. We have leaned heavily on our faith that God would help us through each crisis.

Over the years, I have remembered Marshall's smile and spirit, but it has been my faith and Marcus Jr.'s spirit that has propelled our family through this journey. Marcus Jr. acknowledges that he has sickle cell anemia and that it impacts his life, but he does not let his illness define him. He is a strong, resilient young man. Despite his illness, he is also ever the optimist and genuinely sees the best in others and in life. In fact, he routinely reminds me to "relax" and "not to worry."

In the midst of a sickle crisis, he asks those rhetorical questions and laments the lack of a cure, but he is still a kid, just living. He gets restless after a few days in the hospital and misses his friends. He thinks about all the schoolwork accumulating while he is absent. Yet, he always reminds me not to worry. One of Marcus Jr.'s favorite sayings is, "I got this!" He is correct most of the time. He has it!

Unfortunately, I am not always able to take Marcus Jr.'s advice not to worry. In fact, I worry a lot about his illness, that there have been too few significant advancements in treating or curing sickle cell anemia, and even about the long-term effects of the current treatment options. I also worry about how he will manage the disease into adulthood.

In addition to my worries about his health, I am anxious about his academic performance, even when he is not sick. I think about the challenges he will encounter in life and wonder how he will respond. I worry about whether I am providing him with the skills necessary to thrive as a confident, self-sufficient adult. None of these concerns are related to his illness – they are concerns of a parent.

It might seem odd that in sharing my journey of faith, I would also share my fears and concerns. Worry is a contradiction of faith. In fact, there is an adage about this contradiction: If you pray, why worry? Why pray if you are going to worry? Those of us who profess faith should not worry at all. But fear and worry are not figments of the imagination. In fact, they remain a forever presence.

So, how have I dealt with this issue? I have had to consciously remind myself to be anxious for nothing (Philippians 4:6) and to take everything to God in prayer. A writer, Solly Ozrovech, once wrote that "the love of God expels all fear because the source of fear (and worry), namely sin, was conquered by Jesus."

My "walk in faith" has been and continues to be a journey. Navigating the obstacles with my sons' conception, delivery, and chronic illness has solidified my faith in God. I have needed to draw on my faith in a way that I would have never imagined, particularly when Marcus Jr. has been in sickle crisis. It is hard for a parent to see their child in pain and not be able to provide any relief. That takes another level of faith. I have often found myself crying in the bathroom and asking God for pain relief for Marcus Jr. At the same time, I have prayed for the strength to make it through another night of watching him suffering. I admit that I have wavered in the belief that I had enough faith to sustain me through this journey.

There have been many times when I knew I couldn't continue in my own strength. In these times, I have had to A.S.K. for help. I Acknowledged my feelings, turned to the Source, and then tried to Keep moving. I challenge you to do the same. We are often encouraged to "get over it" when we are "in our feelings." Yet, it is important that we recognize what we are feeling. We should give ourselves time to acknowledge that our feelings are valid. We must also understand the source of our feelings. Most importantly, we must recognize that we have help for our journey.

I know that my concerns about Marcus Jr.'s condition and my weariness after days without sleep are warranted. However, I always feel that I should be able to handle the situation. Why? This is our norm and it could be worse. Over the years, I have learned to give myself a bit of grace. Watching my child suffer in agony, sleeping for only two hours a night, struggling with the decision of whether to give my child a narcotic to manage his pain while balancing the fear of addiction, attempting to ascertain whether his pain dictates additional medical treatment, and not knowing if any of the decisions I have made are accurate – these are *not* normal circumstances. It will always be true that things could be worse. Someone else's situation will always be worse than yours. Nevertheless, it does not lessen the pain you are experiencing.

I am truly relieved that there is a source outside my own strength, a source that I can rely on. Like Zerubbabel in the Bible, we cannot rely on our own strength or power. There are times we have very little strength for the situation we are facing. Whether we are trying to conceive or simply parenting our children, we can "*not* know." We might not know which course we should take, but we must always know that our wisdom and strength come from a source who is all-knowing.

I can attest that God has always been with us throughout our journey. He has been our source of strength. He will also be with you, even in times of uncertainty and crisis. You must simply trust him and the journey.

Chapter Seven

Stepping Out on Faith
It's Your Season

To everything there is a season, and a time to every purpose under the heaven.
(Ecclesiastes 3:1)

This is your season! You may have begun the journey toward parenthood yesterday or ten years ago. Whatever the case may be, I challenge you to embrace THIS as YOUR season.

For some, the first step after marriage is having a baby. Others may decide to wait until the "perfect time." Regardless of your timing, it can be painful and frustrating if things do not go according to plan. That dreaded question becomes a constant reminder of the painful void you possess when you are unable to conceive. You begin to question everything.

It is during this time of uncertainty that you must *"Trust in the Lord with all thine heart and lean not unto our own understanding"* (Proverbs 3:5). Yes, it is a test of your faith. Walking in faith is not easy. It is even more difficult when we expect a quick fix to our problem. Even when the solution does not come as swiftly as we might like, we can have peace during the journey.

We are told that we should "*glory in tribulations also: knowing that tribulation worketh patience; And patience, experience; and experience, hope*" (Romans 5:3-4). It is with this hope that we can stand in faith and expectancy.

> *We (must) continue in faith grounded and settled and be not moved away from the hope of the gospel which ye have heard...* (Colossians 1:23)

In this case, expectancy is a multi-faceted concept. We must view expectancy in terms of God's ability to fulfill our requests and align our thoughts and actions with this belief. Even before you're pregnant, start planning for the baby that you will soon be expecting. One of my major acts of faith and expectancy was to sew a baby blanket prior to my son's conception. I was interested in learning how to sew, and my first project was to make a blanket. I embraced the opportunity and selected a baby pattern. Why not? I would need it soon enough. I had no guarantee that God would fulfill my desire to have a child; I simply expected him to do so. In fact, I would "*continue in prayer and watch in the same with thanksgiving*" (Colossians 4:2). So, I began to prepare. Sewing a blanket was such a small act of faith, but my faith was rewarded. My son used the blanket until he was six. It was one of his favorites. We still have it and will cherish it forever.

One might argue that Marcus' birth was merely happenstance, or that the doctor simply misdiagnosed my medical condition. Frankly, these are reasonable theories and could easily be correct. Whatever the case, "*For this child I prayed; and the Lord hath given me my petition which I asked of him*" (1 Samuel 1:27). I stand on his promise, and just like Hannah, Elisabeth, and others, I believe that he heard my prayer. As I stood praying unto the Lord, he granted my request. In these modern times, we are more inclined to lean toward intellectually and medically sound reasoning and justifications. Nevertheless, I know without question that God is still performing miracles. I "*staggered not at the promise of God through unbelief; but was strong in faith, giving glory to God; and being fully persuaded that what he had promised, he was able also to perform*" (Romans 4:20-21).

Thinking again about Joel Osteen, I wonder, "What would have happened to me, had I not believed?" Step out on faith! Pray and expect that God will answer your prayer. This is your season! If nothing else, know that prayer can position you to hear God. Your path to parenthood may be the result of medical intervention. Your path may be through foster care or adoption. Whatever the route, God possesses the means to carry you there. So, step into the Faith Zone and know that God will answer your prayer!

Chapter Eight

Sustaining Faith

What manner of child shall this be! And the hand of the Lord is with him. (Luke 1:66)

For whom he did foreknow, he also did predestinate to be conformed to the image of his Son, that he might be the firstborn among many brethren. Moreover whom he did predestinate, them he also called: and whom he called, then he also justified: and whom he justified, them he also glorified. (Romans 8:29-30)

Marcus is here! Yet our journey continues. His birth was a testimony of our faith. Addressing the challenges associated with his sickle cell diagnosis is and will continue to be a testimony of our sustaining faith. Despite his diagnosis, we say that Marcus does not have an abnormality. He is one of many, *"for God has created (Marcus) for his glory. He has formed him; yea, He has made him"* (Isaiah 43:7).

Indeed, Marcus was created for God's glory. His birth and diagnosis were only the beginning of understanding our calling. Marcus is the firstborn of a generation that will benefit from the Lampkin family fulfilling God's purpose and plan for our lives. We understand and wholeheartedly believe, *"For unto whomsoever much is given, of him shall be much required"* (Luke 12:47). We were given one of the most truly precious gifts that God can give: the gift of life. We give thanks that Marcus was predestined. We also thank God that he and our work is already justified and glorified. To God be the glory.

Now faith is the substance of things hoped for, the evidence of things not seen.

Hebrews 11:1

Afterword

Dr. Dawnette Y. Banks

In this awe-inspiring work, Dr. Latara and Marcus Lampkin have provided a robust testimonial, chronicling their journey in believing God for the seemingly impossible: the conception and birth of their son, Marcus M. Lampkin Jr. Afforded the blessing of being chosen as Marcus Jr.'s godmother, I took pleasure in coupling my faith with theirs and witnessing the wondrous demonstration of God's power to reward implicit trust in Him with the manifested miracle of life.

I am reminded of Isaiah 53:1, which states, *"Who hath believed our report? and to whom is the arm of the Lord revealed?"* Because we are living in a world systematically characterized by opposing reports and belief systems, it takes a measure of courage and faith to take a stance on any position that is opposed by societal norms. In this scripture, the prophet Isaiah makes a bold inquiry about who would believe the *report of the Lord*, or more explicitly, the message and power of the Messiah, alluding to the fact that both the message and the power of the Messiah would be scarcely credited by most of society during that period. Others in scripture were challenged with this same question. Consider the woman with the issue of blood (Mark 5:25-34), who heard and believed the *report of the Lord*. When doctors had done all they could but could not heal her, she believed and touched the hem of Jesus' garment and was healed. In Romans 4:17-21, Abraham is highlighted as one of the great heroes of faith because he believed the *report of the Lord* that he and his wife Sarah would have a son. Knowing the reproductive limitations of his old age and Sarah's barren womb, Abraham was still convinced that what God promised, He was able to perform.

Similarly, in 2005, Latara and Marcus were faced with the same daring inquiry posed by the prophet, Isaiah, when they received the opposing report from the doctors that they would not be able to conceive a child without medical intervention. Their account is very transparent about the ebb and flow of maturing faith, noting periods when their faith was both challenged and fortified. However, it is evident that God's Word consistently fueled, ignited, and sustained their faith, as this work is masterfully layered with a tapestry of revelatory insight and application of scripture.

I am amazed by and applaud this work's literary craftsmanship in unveiling the heart-stirring inspiration and expository understanding of trusting God for the impossible. This book propels us from strength to strength and glory to glory, as we too face daunting reports that will undeniably place our faith on trial. I am eternally grateful to Latara and Marcus for allowing us to share in their journey so that we can move more confidently forward, embracing future opportunities where our faith will be rewarded in exponential ways!

Dawnette Y. Banks, Ph.D.
Dreamcast Educational Consulting, Owner and CEO

Laurel, Maryland

Acknowledgments

We would like to thank our family and friends who supported us after Marcus' conception, throughout our pregnancy, and during Marcus' initial and subsequent crises associated with sickle cell anemia. To name each of you and your contributions would be an impossible task. Please know that we love and appreciate each of you.

We would like to extend special thanks to our parents, Florence S. Maitland, Gloria J. Williams, James Lampkin (deceased), John H. Osborne Jr., and Rosa Osborne, who, through their faith, unselfish love, and commitment to our growth and development, gave us our first lessons in love and parenthood. We are so blessed that Marcus has the opportunity to experience the love and devotion that only grandparents can give.

Dr. Dawnette Banks (Goddie), Ronald Stephens Jr. (Uncle Ronald), Ricky and Felicia Hammond, we thank each of you for accepting the major responsibility of being godparents to Marcus. Aunts (Kimberly, Karen, Erika, Van, and June) and uncles (John, Timothy, Kenneth, Ronald, Tariun, Nicholas, James Jr., and Tracy), we thank you for what you have done, are doing, and will do in the future to help us nurture and guide Marcus to become all that God has created him to be.

Pastors Kenneth and Nerissa Jackson, thank you for your guidance, prayers, and prophetic words. Pastor and cousin, Nerissa, I am deeply saddened that this work was not completed before you departed to be with the Lord. You were and will always remain a model of a loving mother and wife. Pastor and cousin, Kenneth, you officiated our wedding ceremony in July 2001, and five years later, you christened our son. Your words during that service changed our lives. We have seen the manifestations of your words and have remained excited about ALL that God has in store. We thank God for your ministry.

Regina, my absolute best friend forever, I am so grateful for your lifetime sisterhood, friendship, inspiration, and support. Kay, my other lifetime friend, you too are an inspiration and a true friend, indeed. There will always be an opportunity for a SugarRush because of you! My big sisters, Sonya Lawhorn, Felicia Banks West and Johnetta Colson and my little sisters, Erika Raines, Eulinda Smith, and Sylvia McBurroughs, you have led by example and have been willing to be led by the Holy Spirit. You will always be an inspiration to me. Dr. Tamara Bertrand Jones, my colleague and friend, thank you. Words cannot say how much I appreciate you. "You so pretty," both inside and out! You exemplify the idea of being "true to thine own self." Lynn Comer, my colleague and friend, thank you for your encouragement to move this project forward. I am eternally grateful for you.

We would also like to thank our OPPAGA family, the "caucus." Rashada, Jeanine, Marcus, and Charmetria (one of God's angels on earth, now in heaven), you supported us during our difficult pregnancy. God, we thank you for sharing your angel, Charms, if only for a brief time. Mrs. Cleo, thank you for introducing me to the power of "giving him 40 days."

Dr. Lora Cohen-Vogel (Dan), mentor and dear friend, thank you for committing to my educational and professional development, and most of all, for supporting me in the "midst of many storms." Noah and Benjamin, thank you for sharing your mommy, providing words of comfort, and donating toys that indeed made "baby Marcus feel better" during his hospital visits.

Also, special thanks to Nathan Archer and the members of Team MLJ. We will continue to walk and run to "make awareness and research for sickle cell anemia a priority."

Our current (Florida Center for Reading Research) and former (Educational Leadership and Policy Studies) Florida State University family, we thank you. Amy McKnight, Jimmy Pastrano, and Dr. Patrice Iatarola your support during the early years was invaluable.

Boys Town North Florida family, we thank you for all your support. We pray that you will continue to touch and change the lives of children through your work. In the words of Father Flanagan, we know that "the work will continue, you see, whether (we are) there or not, because it is God's work, not (ours)."

I must acknowledge the ministries that have been my source of inspiration during this journey: Glades Covenant Community Church (Pastor Kenneth Jackson Jr.), Pahokee Deliverance Christian Center (Pastor Willie Hickman Jr.), Bethel AME Church (Dr. Julius H. McAllister Jr.), Potter's House (Pastor T. D. Jakes), and Lakewood Church (Pastor Joel Osteen).

Finally, thank you Marcus M. Lampkin Jr. for being the greatest gift of our lifetime. You are an intelligent, creative, and resilient young man. We pray that the light in your eyes never dims and the love in your heart (for everyone and all things) never fades. We are and will always be your proud parents. Go forth, my son, in confidence knowing that, "You got *this* and God's got you!"

We have much to be thankful for; God is truly worthy to be praised. **To carry out this mission requires enormous effort. To carry out the vision- enormous faith. Yet, the rewards are even greater. To God be the glory!**

Marcus & Latara Lampkin

About the Authors

Latara O. Lampkin, Ph.D. is a research scientist at Florida State University. As an education policy and research scholar, her research spans both K-12 and higher education policy, with a focus on policies and reform efforts designed to increase the educational outcomes for underserved student populations, students in low-performing schools and at minority-serving institutions, particularly Historically Black Colleges and Universities. She is also the owner and CEO of Eduprehd Research and Development Partners, LLC, partnering with non-profit organizations and educational stakeholders to develop, implement and scale-up evidence based programs to increase the educational access and success of under-represented and undeserved students.

Latara writes, researches, teaches, and presents on educational research, policy, and leadership issues used by researchers, practitioners, policymakers, and parents to inform educational decision-making for students in traditional and non-traditional educational settings. She has published work in *American Educational Research Journal, Journal of Leadership and Policy in Schools, Educational*

Evaluation and Policy Analysis, Educational Administration Quarterly, Journal of Negro Education, and *Journal of Research Initiatives,* among other peer-reviewed journals. She has also written several national reports, including those published by the Institute of Education Sciences. This book, *In Faith*, is her most cherished publication and is the inaugural work of the *Faith Rewarded*® series.

Latara serves on the Advisory Board for the Leon County Sickle Cell Foundation, belongs to the National Achievers Society Parent Association (Tallahassee Area Coalition Center of Excellence), and serves on various committees for Boys Town of North Florida. She is also a member of Alpha Kappa Alpha Sorority, Inc. She holds a Ph.D. in Educational Leadership and Evaluation from Florida State University, with a concentration in education policy; a M.A.S.S. in Public Administration from Florida A & M University; and a B.S. in Criminology from Florida State University.

Marcus M. Lampkin, M.S., currently serves as the Executive Director for Boys Town North Florida. Boys Town is a therapeutic treatment program that serves abused and neglected youth.

Marcus' dedication to children and families spans more than two decades. Prior to his appointment as North Florida's executive director, he served in various capacities within the organization and other human service agencies. Marcus holds a Master's of Science degree in Individual and Family Services, and a Bachelor of Science in Criminal Justice with a minor in social work. Marcus currently serves on local, regional, and national committees, advocating for youth and families. Understanding the challenges that social service institutions and systems face when serving youth and families, he continues to seek and implement innovative approaches to enhance family and youth services for children and families of all races and socio-economic backgrounds.

Their Ministry

Marcus and Latara met in 1995 and were joined in marriage in 2001. They are the proud parents of Marcus M. Lampkin Jr. Marcus and Latara are committed to improving the lives of children through research-based programs geared toward addressing the educational, developmental, mental, and social needs of youth and families. They are also committed to empowering families with children diagnosed with sickle cell disease. The have established Team MLJ to support initiatives for the Leon County Sickle Cell Foundation. A portion of the proceeds from their Faith Rewarded® series will be donated to the Sickle Cell Foundation and other organizations engaged in advocacy and research for children with chronic illnesses, in honor of their son, Marcus M. Lampkin Jr. Marcus, Latara and Marcus Jr. reside in Tallahassee, Florida.

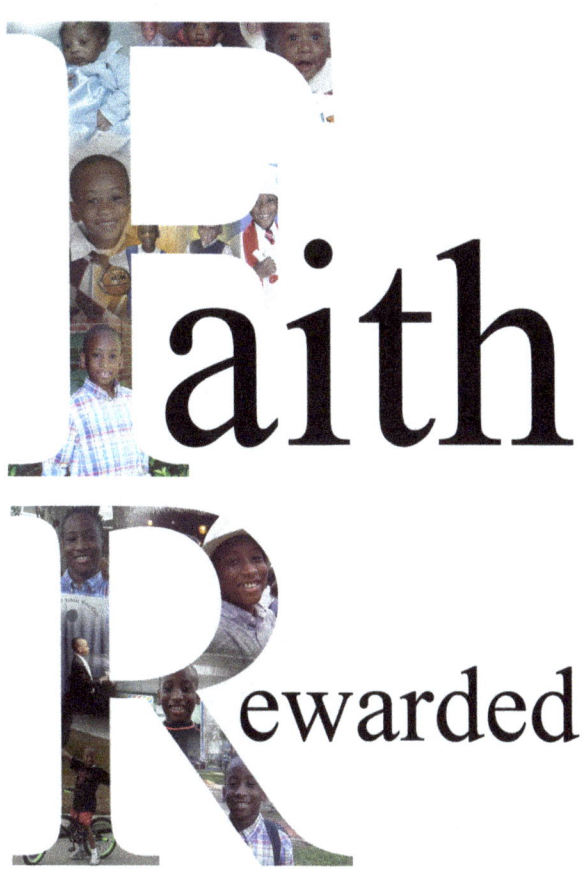

Faith Rewarded

*"If ye have faith as a grain of mustard seed,
...nothing shall be impossible unto you."*

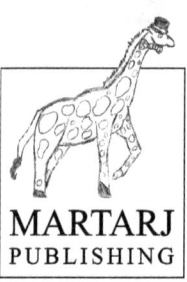

Find more products and
resources at martarj.com.